Caregiving for Beginners

*What I Learned Caregiving for
Frank and his Dementia*

Frank's Wife

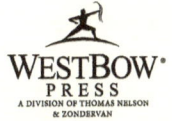

WESTBOW°
P R E S S
A DIVISION OF THOMAS NELSON
& ZONDERVAN

WestBow Press books may be ordered through booksellers or by contacting:

WestBow Press
A Division of Thomas Nelson & Zondervan
1663 Liberty Drive
Bloomington, IN 47403
www.westbowpress.com
1 (866) 928-1240

ISBN: 978-1-4908-4807-5 (sc)
ISBN: 978-1-4908-4806-8 (e)

Library of Congress Control Number: 2014914382

Printed in the United States of America.

WestBow Press rev. date: 10/24/2014

Contents

I've crossed many bridges in my life. The supports under every bridge must be strong or the bridges would collapse.

To: Valerie, Sheila, Mary, Dolly, Francesca, Patti, Dr. Carter and Becky, Dr. Valcour and all the researchers at UCSF, thank you for being my supports.

Introduction

Ok. My first advice for you is to skip this part. Yes, I said skip! There is no need for you to read this little book front to back. Just go to any of the chapters you're having trouble with- read those, skip around, come back here when or if you're ready.

I'm writing this book to hopefully, help you through one of toughest challenges in life you have ever faced. I'm doing it now, because if I can do this- you can too. If I can help even one of you make it through one more day, I'll have succeeded in my humble effort here.

In some of the chapters, I describe my efforts for Frank as he is now (many years after his Dementia began.) Your guy/gal may not be there yet.

Don't let what has happened to Frank's symptoms over a sort of slow motion period of time scare you off. I learned these "skills" over time and you can too.

Another thing you need to know is that my very strong Catholic faith has helped strengthen me and has given me the courage to go on. I don't want you to be put off by my spiritual journey. I know some of you have not strong belief system. I will not try to convert you. I promise. I want you to know that I will do my best here to not sound too "preachy".

I don't want you to be put off by my spiritual journey. I know some of you have no strong belief system. I will not try to convert you. I promise.

My only reason for writing this is that the doctors at the research clinic say Frank's one of the longest living Frontal Temporal Dementia patients they have. They urged me to keep notes and perhaps write something to help other caregivers with little tips and creative ways of caring for a loved one.

I am sure you will wonder about me and my life with Frank. You can turn to Chapter 14-for those details.

Just know that for now- I am here to help you if I can. And to help you keep him/her at home with you for as long as you can. (Longer than you think, if you develop your coping skills.)

My journey these past 8 yrs. has been epic for me. With the help of counseling and my faith I have become a changed person. (I know, for the better) But more about that later. Let's help you now.

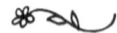

Getting My Head On Straight

After Frank was diagnosed, every morning I'd wake up thinking:" He's going to die. The man I have always loved is going to die!" I was a wreck- you know the drill: can't sleep, can't eat, worried about the kids, worried about finances.......

I began having panic attacks. I went to my doctor when I had what I call "My Target parking lot incident." I was just beginning my errands one spring morning, when I got out of my car: I felt itchy all over and kind of "off". I figured it was allergies and got back into my car, took an antihistamine and waited for the itching to stop. When I looked in the mirror my face looked red and blotchy, like hives. I began to feel a tightening in my chest and knew something was really wrong. I drove like a mad woman over to my doctors, with no appointment. They thought I was having a heart attack- and so did I! After an hour in a dark examining room and an EEG; my doctor came in and told me I was not going to believe this; but I was having an anxiety attack! Me? I know, she said, but here's a prescription for Zoloft and the name of three therapists. I was stunned. I didn't need a therapist- I needed my husband not to have Dementia!

The attacks continued, I lost weight, then decided maybe I needed help from someone, anyone!

Months later, money well spent on a counselor who saved me from myself; I began to understand that Frank wasn't dead yet. I was behaving as though he was. I was grieving before his funeral. I learned I had many more memories to make with him before the end. I could still cherish the man I married; even celebrate what parts of him still remained.

You need to know that I live in a small town. I've taught the little children of this town about God for the past 35 years. Two generations of children have heard me tell them: "God wants you to be happy. He has a path for your life. Finding the path God has for your life is not easy but you will be happiest if you follow His path rather than your own." Now I was lost! What path could I ever take that would make me happy with what I was facing?

The little children (now adults) were watching me. Would I practice what I had preached all these years? I wasn't sure if I could.

Ok. If you think this parts too "preachy" just skip to the next chapter now.

One day the priest at Sunday services in our small church, was telling us about the anniversary of

Our Lady Of Lourdes, in France. He told us of St. Bernadette. I knew the story, but not that she had lived in France. (St. Bernadette is the patron saint of the sick.) Millions of pilgrims have gone to France some have even been cured. We really couldn't afford a trip like that, but I was determined.

With the help of our local priest and a wonderful Irish Pilgrimage Society Group; we traveled to Lourdes in the south of France. This group of sixty, many with health problems, some in wheel chairs, traveled with two young nurses. The group go every year. This is their "vacation". Something like you'd go to Disneyland with your children for a vacation. Many of them are factory workers, or retirees. The faith that bound them together was so strong, it enfolded me and lifted me up. The tens of thousands of Pilgrims in Lourdes that summer marching by candlelight, some on gurneys with nurses pushing them, all singing and praising God and Our Lady of Lourdes -to those who don't know - is Mary, mother of Jesus. It is said that the waters that spring from the Grotto have cured hundreds. I brought some home in little bottles for my friends and relatives. Frank and I drank from the waters.

Frank and I did whatever the Lourdes pilgrims from Ireland did. Frank asked me after few days:

"Why are we going to Mass every day?" He didn't understand how devout these people were. Neither did I, until I had been with them staying at the same hotel, listening to their troubled stories, singing with them, eating with them, for a week.

And like a sponge, I absorbed the combined prayer and the faithful "cloud" surrounding these special people. Thousands of faithful people. I had gone to France looking, hoping for, a "miracle" for Frank. But I came home with a small "miracle" for myself. I had found the path God wanted for me to take, the one that really would make me the happiest. And I was determined to follow it well.

I discovered that if I could find creative ways to help care for Frank, I would be following God's path. Oh, of course I have my bad days, days I wish- I don't know- this time could be past, but then I wouldn't have any of Frank left. I am not willing to give him up not until God decides the turn of the path.

And so my friends: that's how I got my head on straight!

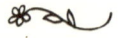

Traveling With Frank

At first, when Frank was diagnosed, I was devastated. My thoughts ran to: "We'll never travel again! We had such plans! Poor me, poor me, poor us, poor us." I soon discovered (with help from my counselor) that life did not have to be over. With a little imagination, I could still make memories with Frank. Good memories.

We went on day trips. We went over night to the ocean. We went to Oregon to visit our niece and her family. We went to San Diego to visit our other niece. We even traveled to France! When we were in Paris, I will always remember our small hotel. You could lean out the window and see the Eiffel Tower. The tower has little white lights all night; but just after 9:00pm the French put on a light show. Beautiful! Frank wouldn't go to bed while we were there, until after he saw the show.

I tried to plan for any eventuality. I made sure I had plenty of identification for Frank; both on his body and in his wallet. I had current pictures of him in my wallet. I did "lose" him in a department store several times. (He was constantly in search of a bathroom.)

But the great memories I have of our trips, outweigh the fearful moments. These memories are, for me, worth everything.

It took me awhile to figure out that he was having trouble holding his urine until he found a bathroom. (Looking back, I guess he was visiting every rest stop and bathroom just to make sure he didn't wet.) This came clear to me once, when he returned, after trying to get to a bathroom. He was walking bowlegged and wet clear down to his socks! Then I understood. I went to Costco and bought depends for him. I never discussed it. I just gave his regular underwear away and substituted the depends. I always call them "his underwear" and he doesn't object.

There did come a time when even side by side with me in the grocery store, he would just walk ahead of me and do "his walk about" in the store. This will happen to you too. It's almost as though his childish wish to "be on his own" makes him walk a little faster! The worry makes for a stressful trip to town. But I still do it. It's part of my life now and I won't let Frank's Dementia clip our wings.

I have a widow friend who comes once a week; that way I can have him stay at home while I get time consuming errands done.

Don't waste anytime now; make new memories to outweigh the sad ones.

You just have to plan and know you can do it! If I did, then you can too!

How to Deal With "Helpful" and Not So "Helpful" Family and Friends

I used to get defensive with my relatives when they called or visited and questioned me about Frank. I thought they were in some way judging my care giving practices and decisions. It frustrated me until I finally realized that they were grieving for Frank as much as I was. They were expressing their worry and advice, "helping" in their own way. I finally realized that all the advice, etc. was just an expression of love and wanting to "help."

Now I listen with a different attitude. I accept that they care. I listen and reassure them how much I appreciate their advice. I tell them, if I can, that their advice is a good idea that I might try. That makes them feel part of the care giving. I try not to get too "into" Frank's everyday decline: it will usually result in a statement like "Oh, this is just too much for you; you need to put him in a nursing facility!" My answer to that is usually to brush this aside with: "This is my journey and I'm coping and taking care of myself. I love taking care of him (even if it's not really true on that particular day.) I wouldn't have it any other way."

Don't be embarrassed or hesitant in telling your family and friends what you need in the way of support. True friends and family will be supportive, but may need to be schooled in helping you. You're the teacher in this area; just be as gentle as you can.

You can also say that what you need is their continued support and caring, but not so much advice.

You'll find that some friends make you feel worse and some make you feel better after you've talked to them. My rule of thumb has been to stay in contact more often with people who "help" you feel stronger. Limit your contact with the others.

This is a very isolating journey. It will help you to unburden to one or two people. Your unhappiness and fear will overwhelm you at times. That's why, if you can afford it, I suggest a counselor be one of those people you unburden to.

I also want to tell you about a mistake I made at the very beginning of Frank's illness. When he could be left without someone watching him, to keep him safe: I didn't seek out the Alzheimer's group in my area. They have meetings regularly and I thought I lived too far away to travel at night to any meetings. I should have made more of an effort. They could have helped me feel less isolated and given me valuable advice at the <u>beginning.</u> Business advice is one of the areas you'll need to get advice for. See more about this in the chapter on "Dealing with Finances and other "Do it yourself" projects.

Keeping Frank Safe at Home and Abroad

Frank and I went to a Christmas Day family gathering at a dear friend's house. There were children going in and out all the doors of the living room and kitchen. (Five doors in all.) I stationed myself near the front door- Frank could easily go out all four of the back doors leading to the backyard, so I figured my spot kept him from getting into the street and of course, lost.

Well unfortunately the side gate between the driveway and the backyard was not in repair. Actually it was not there at all! So the entire afternoon I was watching backyard doors, front door, and trying to relax and enjoy the company of my friends and family.

Frank doesn't just wander -he walks fast, even faster when he feels he's getting "away". Family and friends were so good; they helped me by alerting me and/or getting Frank when he was outside. After a few hours of this I was so exhausted that I made my early goodbyes, went home and napped, while Frank did his "walkabout" in the relative safety of our house.

Making your home as "safe" as you can will help you find time to relax and renew for the times when you must wake yourself up at night or untangle your guy or gal from some dangerous situation they've managed to get into.

I started by getting very inexpensive "child proof" doorknob covers from Toys'R Us. My doorknobs are round and the covers fit perfectly. I put them on all the outside doors. (Of course Frank had had to "get lost" outside a few times before I did this.) It's safer if you deal with this first thing.

The second thing I did was hire a carpenter to put in some "childproof gates". (If you have a one story house this is not necessary.) I have a tri-level house that just screamed- "he'll fall down the stairs!" I had the carpenter put the gates at the bottom of one set of stairs and the top of the other set.

The idea was to make a "safe" one level area that he could walk to his heart's content. My home has an open living room-dining room and kitchen. He loves to walk in a circle around and around. It keeps him active and entertained.

Safety proofing the kitchen was a tough one. But I just attached a huge wide very long black elastic to one of the cabinet knobs and then to the door to the deck. It acts as a visual reminder to him to stop. It works most of the time. Other times he gets so engrossed in the stretchy fabric and tying it to other kitchen knobs, that he doesn't bother to enter the kitchen area.

If you can, install a child-gate to the kitchen. Installing child proof knobs on the stove, is also advisable.

Frank also likes to turn the lights on and off. I try not to be irritated by these things. He wouldn't do this before (he always turned off lights to save energy before his Dementia.) He also likes to turn water off and on in the sinks. I just make sure the hot water in the single faucet handle is turned to cold. I can hear the water running even when I'm in another part of the house. I turn off a lot of water faucets.

You'll find that (as with any small child) they'll figure some other way to get your heart pounding with adrenaline.

Another, very important task for keeping Frank safe was to send away for a bracelet or have one made that has his name, medical condition, phone numbers, even doctor's name and number on it. At first Frank wouldn't wear the bracelet, so I just got him to wear the necklace. It looks like a Saint Christopher medal. Later though it was easier to get him wear both. It gives me a sense that if we're ever separated in town, someone will know who to call. (My cell phone number's is on his bracelet.)

Sometime later; I installed toilet rails on each of our toilets. It was easier for me to verbally direct him to the handles to get him seated on the toilet. They work pretty nice for me too!

I can't say this enough to you: This happened over many months and there is no need to stress about the timing. You'll know and see the need for more safety.

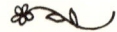

Keeping Frank Clean-The Water Wars

A funny thing happens with dementia patients. They don't like water (especially when it involves bathing.) The sound of it, the feel of it; makes bath time and face washing a real challenge. I try to give Frank a shower every other day. Having a clean smelling loved one makes you want to kiss and hug him and really helps with keeping his skin healthy.

I ALWAYS sing to him in the shower. I even start to hum when we are getting ready to get in. I get down to my undies and help him in the shower. This helps me to test the water on my legs and helps to calm him. I try to work my way up from his toes to his face and hair. (Doing face and hair last seems to work best since that's the time he objects to the most.) I sing little children's songs all during his shower. I've evolved to a shower chair, with me behind him singing.

With a little imagination and trial and error, bath time can be work for you but happy for him/her.

Drying him in winter is tough. He gets the shakes really easily. So I purchased a terry bathrobe. I put it next to the shower. After his shower I put that on him then dry his hair with a towel just as fast as I can. (I think that dementia patient's bodies have a hard time adjusting body temperature.) So I try extra hard to dry him as quickly as I can. If he wants to walk and won't stand still I just direct him to touching the towel rack or some other object to hold his attention (while singing the whole time.) I ask him to look for the blue dots that I've placed in the shape of a hand (on the shower wall.) That gets him to focus on something and keep his feet still while you dress him/her.

I try to shave him after I get him dressed. (He has a tough beard and the steam from the shower really makes it easier to shave him.) Boy did I have to teach myself how to shave a man! I had no idea what a chore this is for men everywhere! I try to make shaving a happy time for him by sitting him down in front of the dining room window, so he can look out at the birdfeeder when I shave him. And as they say: "practice makes perfect." The good news is: that something that used to take me 1 hour, now take 20 minutes! Hurray for economy of motion! Sometimes I shave him every other day, so as not to irritate his skin.

Lucky for me, Frank became urinary incontinent about a year before his bowels failed him. It took me awhile to "get it". That first year before his urinary incontinence was full blown; it was "Where's the nearest bathroom?" On trips of even half an hour, he was constantly asking "Where's the bathroom?" When we traveled on longer trips in the car we had to stop at every rest stop, adding hours to our travel time and really annoying me. Finally, when he'd completely wet himself – I "Got it!" I went to Costco and bought Depends.

Boy, what did our grandparents do without Depends? I took them home and always called them "underwear". I did have to experiment with the correct size. I bought too big at first and he wet right down the sides. (Snug is better.) I gave away his regular underwear and put these in his drawer. I still call them his underwear.

I ended up having to "water proof" all the chairs where he likes to sit. But if I'm not lazy about checking and changing him every few hours, the pads on the chairs stay dry. I try not to blame him when there's a "wet slip". It's not his fault, but mine. I sing a little song when I change him and try hard never to sound annoyed. He can't help this and would toilet himself, if he could. (Sometimes when he first started this, I know he was ashamed and embarrassed.) So I try never to admonish him, just make up a song like: "This is the way we change your undies, this is the way we change your undies." You'll know it's worth it when you see him/her smile. I also use baby powder to keep him comfortable and smelling nice.

On to the changing of depends and the dreaded "bowel movement"!

PLEASE! Don't go any further until you need to. (Too much information!)

★★★★★★★★★★★★★★★★★★★★★

I think changing Frank's depends, when he has a bowel movement, is the hardest thing I've ever had to "creatively" do. Just the smell is off-putting. I had to really develop my skills on this one! First, in the bathroom, with him in tow (speaking or singing softly puts him at ease.) I close the door and stop <u>breathing through my nose!</u> Whenever I forget and smell, I blame myself not him.

Next I am prepared, prepared. BEFORE I remove any of his cloths! I have purchased disposable latex gloves (Boxes of them in each bathroom.) and sturdy baby wipes. (Also a box in each bathroom.) Same goes for depends and a pair of blunt nosed scissors–placed out of sight under the wipe box.

I put the <u>gloves on first</u>, after closing the bathroom door. Talking softly, or singing, to him all the time; I pull up one arm of his shirt above the elbow and fold it into the neck of his shirt. I'm trying to enfold his one

20

arm in the shirt. (This, so I can keep his shirt clean and dry without removing it and keep his one hand from interfering, ugh, with my cleaning.) Next I direct his one hand to hold onto the sink rim, then take off his shorts or pants <u>only</u>. One leg at a time, I remove them. When it's just me breathing thru my mouth and he in his depends, I walk him into the shower. I can stay outside on this one. I then direct him to touch and see the blue dots. I've put blue dots in the shower so he's facing in the direction I need him to be. He's, hopefully, keeping his free hand occupied with the blue dots. Then using the blunt nosed scissors, I cut his smelly depends on each side, deftly catching and wiping the bowel movement as I remove his depends. This all can go smoothly or messily. Just keep trying to perfect your "skills". The depends can also be torn easily at the seams on each side. (Good to know if you're ever without scissors!)

When his depends are off and placed out of the shower, I use baby wipes to get the most that's left on him. Sometimes, if it's enough (I don't have to shower him from the waist down.) Sometimes it's a mess. When that happens I just turn the hand held shower on, adjust the water temp, and with soap and warm water get the job done. No breathing allowed!

Keeping him/her clean and dry is truly important. Sores or breaks in their skin can easily lead to infection and doctors' visits. Frank's skin has become very sensitive to everything-hot, cold, certain topical creams, even pressure from sitting or leaning for short periods of time. (Not at all like our skin would react.)

Remember, you can try anything new that I haven't thought of. You may even do a better job than I- just keep trying.

Now, back to the Water Wars: I used to have to change the sheets and waterproof mattress protectors in the middle of the night. It made me grumpy. Now it's easier for me to change; even if he wets through the "first line of protection."

My "first line of protection" is a small 36x36 water proof quilted pad with two layers of towels on top.

I've learned that when Frank sleeps he is more relaxed and he'll urinate over a single pad during the night. So, I put two layers of bath towels: which consist of two hand towels and one bath towel- works best for my washing machine. Putting two sets of wet towels and two pads is all I put in my washer, otherwise the heavy towels will make the machine go off center. I prepare three dry individual sets of pads for the night. One more thing I've done: invested in two really good waterproof mattress protectors. Those are my "last lines of protection".

Every once in a while, during the night, Frank will move out of position and wet through the towels and pads. I'd have to change the sheet and sometimes the waterproof mattress protector. All I have to do now is just change the extra mattress protector, and sheet and all is well again. I also put an old waterproof pad between the sheet and the mattress cover. After a while the pads wear out and don't hold liquid well. I make sure to mark any of these worn pads with a permanent marker. I have mixed them up in the past and it's a wet mess! I used the marked pads between the sheet and the mattress protector. Just one more line of defense!

I try not to talk in a grumpy voice during my night time changing. I just reassure Frank how much I love him and that I know it's not his fault. (Even if I am grumpy- I don't show it.) Your voice and loving gentle actions will make him/her feel safe and calmer. Again, you may not feel gentle and loving all the time, just pretend, it's well worth it and you'll have less guilty feelings at the end of the day.

Once again I want to emphasize that these efforts to care give for Frank have developed over time, in slow motion. You won't have to use some of these "hints" for many years to come or not at all. You can just come back and read my "hints" when you need them.

Ok. Back to the changing. Now he's dried and with fresh "underwear" on, dressed and ready to go......
Go? Go? What do you do for the rest of the day?

We'll get to that in the chapter "Keeping Frank Stimulated." Just stick with me.

Bedtime

Frank usually walks around in the evenings. (I call this his "walkabouts") It's good exercise and I'm used to it. I've also found it so much better for me to make some time for "me". So I go upstairs around 8:00pm. (I have gates at the bottom of the stairs to keep him downstairs.) I go upstairs, closing the gate, then I brush my teeth, take a shower and get his night-time pills ready. I put out his pajamas and ready the bed with a water proof pad for his side of the bed... (And believe me it's a challenge when they become incontinent.)

I go back down stairs until 9:00pm. I make sure the outside doors are locked. I take Frank by the hand, turn out the lights, and -singing little songs like: 'This is the way we go to bed, go to bed.' (To the tune of "Mary had a little Lamb.") we slowly go up to bed. The singing is very valuable. It makes him less anxious about bedtime. Try to remember that every night is a new experience, a new bedtime in a dark he has never known before.

Upstairs now, I give him his night pills. I keep these in an upstairs drawer. I brush his teeth, singing "this is the way we brush our teeth, etc." With practice you'll get better at brushing. As you become less of an elephant in the china closet, you'll find it much easier. Frank was much more co-operative about opening his mouth, when I was less hurtful, and more skilled. Another tip: I fill the rinse glass with water, wet the brush, and then TURN off the running water. (Again, I discovered the sound of water disturbs him!) I brush his teeth BEFORE I change his depends. Seems the running water sometimes makes him go and I have to change him again. You can read more about the importance of teeth brushing in the chapter: "Hair, Nails, Toes and Teeth".

When I've brushed his teeth I have him sit on the toilet to change him one last time before bed. I have learned that taking his clothes off is much harder than putting them on. So, while he's seated, I try taking his shirt off. His body is lower than mine at this point. So I can pull his shirt over his shoulders and his head as I ask him to bend his head down. This seems to be easier than anything else I've tried. Then I put his pajama tops on (which I have cut short to above his waist.) No pajama bottoms, saves me having to change bottoms during the night, and most of the time the shorter tops stay dry.

I have already readied his side of the bed with the water proof pad set. I was surprised how little liquid one waterproof pad will hold. Frank seems to wet more at night when he's relaxed, than in the day time; the extra towels on top really absorb and I have less chance of a "spill over." You may think of something better. Just use your creative self!

I lead him to the bed and, using a small stepping stool that I've moved next to the bed, I have him step up and I ease him into the exact position I need him to be: over the water proof pad. I'll talk gently to him now, telling him what we are doing, having him give me his elbow so I can lie him down. (I do all this because he's forgotten how to get in bed and it helps calm him for sleep.) I turn on the TV with the sound down low and the timer set to turn off in an hour.

Then I pull the heavy bedroom chair next to him in bed and wedge it into place with a 4X4 I've had cut to the exact space between the chair and the wall. (This last seems to work better than any bed gates I've purchased in the past) Then I activate the little alarm I have, and put it just outside the bedroom door. I purchased it in the Alzheimer's catalogue on line. Costs no more than $40.00 and well worth your getting a somewhat worry free night's sleep.

Then I drink a big glass of water and take a mild sleep aide (your doctor can recommend for you) I get in bed next to him. I get very close, touching him with my arm and we say our prayers. The reason I drink water is, it acts like a timer for me to wake up during the night and go. When I'm up, I check Frank. He's usually wet and I change him and his pad. I don't like him be wet more than four hours and this works for me.

I've found that by using a little imagination, I can put his fresh depends around his ankles first, while he is prone, then, using a blunt pair of scissors, I can cut off his wet depend, wipe him down, then have him standup, as I pull his wet depends back then wrapping the depends and wet pad together, I slip a fresh pad in its place, pull up his new depends then lay him back down. I've learned to do this in a smooth motion. Sounds complicated, but you'll get better at this in time. I also prepare two waterproof pads with towels before going to bed so I can have them handy when I am half asleep. (Easier for me.)

I used to walk Frank to the bathroom to change him. All that did was wake us both up. The above idea turns out to be much easier and we can go back to sleep. (I still have to turn on the TV for a while.) Sometimes I use earplugs during this part of the night.

Lack of sleep is the one thing that makes you irritable, short tempered and a dangerous daytime driver. If you need to sleep in another bedroom (and I've done this sometimes too) don't feel bad. Just remember to put on the room alarm and take the bell part with you to the other room. I also find that cat naps during the day help.

I'll bet you can come up with even better ideas and short cuts than I have. Just use your imagination and creative skills. I've found that I feel less helpless and more loving to Frank when I blame myself if something goes awry, instead of him. I just make a mental note to do it another way next time.

What used to take forty minutes to ready him for bed now takes fifteen minutes. This "economy of motion" is my key to staying committed. It helps me to feel less tired when waking up to a new day.

I tell people that when I wake in the morning, and make care giving for Frank my primary goal: "It's what gets me out of bed in the morning." I feel this is my reason for living now. I'm hopeful you'll feel this way very soon.

Breakfast, Lunch and Dinner

When Frank first was diagnosed I made a real effort to keep him as healthy as I could. This meant to me: healthy regular meals at regular times of the day.

Breakfast sometimes is dependent upon his waking. Since he was a farmer we usually got up around five. But since he takes meds to sleep, he sleeps in until 8:00am or 9:00 am. I get him up, then wash his face, comb his hair and get him bathed or dressed.

You may not need to do any of this at first. It's been several years and taken his slowly diminishing abilities for me to need to do this now.

Anyway back to breakfast. I fix his favorites and sometimes he'll tell me what he wants to eat.

In the first years of his Dementia, he would eat very fast. We used to joke that "Grandpa was the first to want dessert, because he eats so fast!" He gained quite a bit of weight those years, which was very unlike him as he had always watched his weight and never weighed more than five pounds over his normal weight.

His tastes also changed. He liked sweets more; to the point where I had to hide the dinner dessert until after he finished his main meal. I went along with the taste changes as long as he got a well-rounded, 3-5fruits & vegetables, 6 oz. of protein and 6-8 8oz glasses of water a day. Breads and dessert are always optional.

Now he eats more slowly and he's back to his normal weight. He even eats so slowly that I've bought an hour glass and set it on the table within his sight. I turn it when he sits down and now, as he seems to be more aware of time passing, he eats at a better pace.

Something I have discovered: Dementia patient's sense of time is distorted. I couldn't figure if time was moving slower for Frank or faster. I finally over time, observed that time moves slower for him: When he walks slowly, he thinks it's his normal pace. If I move quickly to give him a kiss or help him with a step down, he flinches. I try to imagine if things came at me at 10 times faster than I expected, I'd flinch too!

Lunch is usually at noon. But if he oversleeps in the mornings I just either skip breakfast or do lunch or vice-versa. I also skip any meds that would go with the meal he's skipped.

He does his "walk about" and sometimes his puzzles. We'll talk about games and puzzles in the "Keeping Frank Busy and Stimulated Chapter."

Dinner is usually at 6:00pm

One thing I've had to deal with, which you may not ever, is that in the last year he has taken to getting up after a few bites and walking around the table, even forgetting he's eating a meal. I have solved this for myself by fashioning a cloth belt to tie him gently to his dining room chair. I must caution you: this is not allowed in a licensed care facility and you must do this only for the hour of a meal at home. I know some would call this abuse, but if it is done just until he's eaten enough to be a meal, it works for me. I do sit down with him and remind him to "keep eating dear."

This last device has helped me to keep him safe (otherwise he was picking up a full glass of milk or juice and wandering around with it.) This also has kept me even tempered when I have seen a great meal go to waste or become too cold to eat. Just use your best judgment here and do this lovingly and with a happy voice.

Voices. That reminds me, I have developed a certain voice with Frank. Do you remember the voices you've heard coming from teachers of small children or young parents or even yourself when your children were young? I now talk to Frank in this way and tone. For some reason, it soothes him, makes him feel safe and less anxious. It also has made him more co-operative. Try it, even if it's exhausting at first. It has worked wonders for me.

Now for the eating out in restaurants. I do this occasionally when we must or on special birthdays or anniversaries with friends and family. You can do this too; with a little preparation.

I pack a small bag with a change of clothes, several depends, wipes, a plastic bag, one or two coloring books or puzzles and colored pens. I take the bag to town when I go with Frank. I try hard not to forget it. I take it into the restaurant with me. If I have to go to the bathroom, I do this first: I take him with me into the ladies room, saying "I have to go to the bathroom now and you know how much I like you to hold my hand when I go." We go into the handicapped stall and he holds my hand most of the time. (This prevents any bolts for the door.)

When the waitress comes to seat us I'll ask for a booth or a table next to a wall. I have Frank sit in the both first, then I slide in next to him on the same side. Or if it's a table, I have him sit next to the wall with me next to him. In this way I block any chance of his leaving the table and I have no need to use anything to restrain him. (If you have a similar booth-wall arrangement at home you might not need a belt ever.)

You will be surprised at how helpful and understanding people are when you are out in public.

Don't become a recluse because you are ashamed. I was at first, but have adjusted and we have a great time. I don't do much in the way of shopping when I'm with him. Just marketing and banking. I wait until I can have a neighbor or a helper watch him at home for the time consuming shopping and errands.

You might feel guilty and or relieved the first few times you leave him/her. That's natural. Just get your errands done and try not to worry about him/her. After a while you'll feel better about their well-being and you'll relax.

Doing some things for yourself by yourself is a good way to get out and change your perspective on your daily care giving. I sometimes will make arrangements to have lunch with a friend. It's nice.

Keeping Frank "Stimulated and Busy" Day by Day

Alright, you've got him/her clean, fed, shaved, dressed, and safe; what now?

First, please don't be discouraged when I write anything here that seems years away for you. (I thought I couldn't do this one more week–let alone year after year!) Just take it one day at a time, as they say. OK?

1. <u>Chores around the house.</u> In the first few years he helped with the vacuuming (did a great job); he made the bed with me, prepared meals with me, raked leaves with me, and gardened with me. See where I'm going? Supervised chores were a help to me and a great way to keep Frank busy.

2. <u>Games and cards</u>. The first few years we played games, etc. He was still sharp then. Colorful games seemed to stimulate him the most. (I'd let him win and then praise him.) Just the interaction will help him/her and bring you closer. As for the types of games, go with

your knowledge of yourself and him/her. For instance I bought games that had cars or racing involved since that what he always enjoyed before.

3. <u>Busy by himself</u>. He always liked numbers, so I went to Wal-Mart and got math books, coloring books and mazes for him. (They were about sixth grade level.) He loved solving the problems and spent hours doing even complex division problems. (This changed overtime and I had to buy earlier grades, even preschool math books and mazes, as his abilities declined.)

4. <u>Puzzles. </u>I started out by setting up a card table in the living room with 500 piece puzzles. He enjoyed them but was more patient with the 250 piece puzzles. Then of course this became the simpler wooden toddler puzzles (ten pieces or less.) I still keep them on the counter and every so often he'll stop and put a few pieces in place. I try always to praise him when that happens, then I undo the puzzle when he's gone onto something else. There will come a time when he/she will become less interested in coloring or doing puzzles. (Doesn't seem to do things on his own.) I try to take a few minutes every

day to encourage him with puzzles. Staying stimulated for as long as he can helps his mind stay active.

5. <u>Drawing and painting</u>. One of the doctors mentioned that Dementia patients sometimes become very artistic. So I bought a few canvases, some beginning acrylic colors, and brushes. I set it all up. (Protecting the floor and anything else I needed to cover.) I had him look at a few pictures to give him some ideas and I just let him paint! (I did stay around to supervise any messes.) You should see what he painted! For a man who never ever was interested in art; he painted the most incredible picture! I will keep it always. Sadly, his "artistic period" stopped after that first picture. He did go on to pencil drawing and just plain scribbling, but never picked up a brush again. Perhaps this won't be true for your guy/gal. But I hope you get the idea about "experimenting" with untapped interests.

6. <u>Music</u>. Frank has always loved music. Especially from the 50's and 60's. He even remembers the words to some of the songs and sings along with the music. I'll put an old tune on the CD

and we'll dance along. (He was always a good dancer.) Even now, some old friend will call and ask: "Are you still dancing?" And -yes we are!

7. <u>Exercise and biking</u>. Early on we'd take hikes in the woods, or go biking, not far, but enough to get our adrenaline flowing. Frank also liked to exercise on our stationary bike. He seemed to want to go forever, so I would time him and then "help" him to get off. (Distraction is a great way to get him off and on to thinking about something else.) He can be very focused on something and not want to stop. I sometimes will offer food as an incentive for him to get onto something else. I caution you here: use a patient voice and those creative skills to get him/her to agree to follow your direction. Anger at these times only frightens or confuses them and you will have a stubborn child on your hands.

8. <u>Fix-it Jobs</u>. Early on, when he didn't need much supervision, I'd keep him busy with little simple fix-it jobs. After a while I discovered that he was dangerous to any project and I hid the tools from him. We did do projects together though. We painted the exterior of the house- with

more paint on us than on the house I think. But it was a good thing to do outdoors and together. We even crawled under our old cabin and reinforced the foundation. (That's when I really learned how to pour cement, use power tools and get dirty!) All valuable lessons for me.

Just do what you can and learn what you can so you can remember for them when they no longer can.

You can do it!

9. <u>Sedentary relaxing</u>. Now that time has passed and taken its eventual toll; he likes to watch old western movies, CSI, Bones, Law and Order- but you know your guy/gal best and can figure this out. I've programmed the TV for captioning. He likes to read the captions out loud. It used to bother me, but now I know it's good for stimulating his brain.

10. <u>Traveling and Talking</u>. Whenever we are in the car I play his music and talk to him. I ask him about what we see when we pass a field or a business. He likes to read the signs, even now. Once when we took our regular trip to San Francisco, he kept repeating UPS, UPS, for miles and miles. I finally realized he was

reading the back of the UPS truck in front of us! I also to this day, ask him what color things are. He still knows his colors!

11. <u>Frank's Busy Bag.</u> I've mentioned this before, but bears repeating. Frank has never liked waiting in line. Even more so after his Dementia presented itself. So, I try to plan, plan, plan. I gathered some colored pencils, coloring books, and simple math books from Wal-mart. I keep them in a bag, along with a change of "underwear." I carry this busy bag where ever I go. Keeping it in the car is also a good idea. With his busy bag, he's much more willing to wait at the restaurant, a doctor's office, the DMV etc.

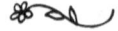

Pills and Meds

This will be a short chapter because I'm not a doctor. Your family doctor will be your best advisor for medications. (Neurologists will have input too, but it's best to have one doctor to advise you and write prescriptions.)

My goal when talking to any doctors about meds: has been:

1. To keep Frank medicated just enough to help him adjust to all the new things he encounters every day. (Adjusting to his level of anxiousness: He's both fearful and restless almost all of his waking hours.) Your guy/gal may have other behavior challenges for you. Meds can help.

2. Medicating Frank ONLY enough to keep him calm and safe; BUT not so much that he sleeps all day or is less active during the day.

This is a fine line for you and your doctor.

My best advice for doing this is to keep a small little note book and enter in it, each day, the meds you have given him/her. Be sure and enter any change in behavior too. (Weak, Dizzy, too sleepy, etc.)

A day or two before your doctor's appointment write down a summary of the meds you've given him/her and any behaviors and/or questions you have. This can help the doctor to evaluate his patient and you won't leave anything of importance out.

Take the booklet and the summary with you to your appointments with any of your doctors. Don't be shy about keeping in touch with him if you think you are overmedicating. (Some people have a sensitivity to regular doses of a medicine; they may need a lesser dose- especially at first.)

Also buying a seven day pill minder, with parts for four times a day dividers, is a great help. It helps me to know when I need to get a refill on any meds a full week in advance. (When you're filling the pill box, you'll notice how little you have left for the next fill time.) Then you can note if any of the meds have no refills left, so you can call the doctor's office in plenty of time. It also helps me to see if I have given or not given a dose. Best thing I have bought for so little money at a drugstore or Wal-Mart.

One more thing about meds. I have found that especially at night, I have trouble getting Frank to swallow his pills. He's tired and I'm tired -it's a struggle. I bought a pill crusher and use a tablespoon and a bit of water and he gets them right down now. Some people use applesauce or pudding instead of water. (Much easier.) Be sure and talk to your doctor -some pills can't be crushed.

Keep trying; you'll get that "economy of motion", I've talked about. When you've figured out the smoothest easiest way of accomplishing a task, it'll take you less time and you'll have more energy for fun things.

You can do this!

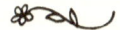

Dealing With Finances and other "Do it Yourself Stuff"

At first it felt weird to begin making decisions all by myself. (I was the less dominant in making business decisions and the purchases of big items.)

I felt adrift when things came up: like who's going to unclog the sink, screw a screw, hammer a nail, or in the case of males; who'll cook, sew a button, do the laundry, iron my shirts?

The answer for me was to learn how to do the things Frank always did, both large and small. It gave me a feeling of strength and satisfaction when I (not so perfectly) completed a challenging chore. I just took it day by day, chore by chore.

One of the big things I had to do was plan for the future. (Just when I was taking little baby steps and learning NOT to look too far ahead.)

Finances were always shared by Frank and I. We discussed various plans and ideas. But he always made the final decisions. I was active and paid the business' bills, but only after he'd OK'd them. So I knew a little bit about our finances. If you don't, you'll have to learn now. Don't put this off. That would be a mistake!

I expected I'd have advice from my friends and family. You will too. Listen to what they have to advise; but think about it and choose how you want to proceed. Don't let yourself be frightened or cajoled into any decisions not your own. No one should push you to make decisions. Early on you and your spouse should discuss financial plans. If at all possible take only your loved one to any meetings with a lawyer. Taking a sibling or child will give too much of your power over to them. You can do it!

I used our lawyer to get our wills in order and on his advice, had written proof from a neurologist that Frank was still in his right mind enough to sign over Power of Attorney and other papers. Our lawyer wanted us to visit the doctor the same day we signed over the final papers. We asked the neurologist for a letter stating Frank's abilities and our lawyer kept the letter with the wills. That way he said, we had proof for our heirs and there'd be less likelihood of any contested wills.

I also had a funeral representative come to the house to discuss and make arrangements for our funerals. (I know, I know, too much to bear.) But, surprisingly, the young man was very informative and kind. We made decisions in a calm unhurried way. We even pre-paid for the future costs of our funerals. I felt so relieved after he left. I have new found respect for people who lose a loved one unexpectedly and have to make these decisions at such an emotional time.

I also decided that I needed a list of relatives and friends and their phone numbers handy to call, or ask a friend to call, personally, when Frank did die. I put this along with his obituary-date left blank of course-in with copies of the funeral arrangements. I put these all together and told one of my children where all this was.

None of the above was easy. It left me drained and shaky. But I persevered.

After I had thought through and done as much pre-planning as possible; I forgot about the future and concentrated on just taking care of Frank. I was surprisingly less burdened.

I'd like to stop here and explain why I am so generic in my descriptions of what I did to get where I am today.

A friend, upon reading the first draft of this, used the word "brutal" to describe some of my explanations. I just want you to know that there were plenty of well-meaning sensitive people saying such consoling things to me in the beginning and even today, upon learning of my current life situation. These wonderful people did not know that their <u>accumulated</u> sympathy for me just made it harder to become the strong person I seem to be today.

I know you will have all the sympathy you will need and more from those around you. I am speaking to you today to help you be strong and not become consumed by your grief. OK? Good!

Today, I take one day at a time and try not to look too far ahead. To be near sighted in life is much better emotionally.

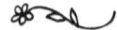

Hair, Nails, Toes and Teeth

Frank had fairly "normal" behaviors for several years. That meant we could get his hair cut at a regular salon or barber shop. There finally came a time when he wouldn't sit still or was "confused" by the people and lights. He just seemed uncomfortable. By that time, I was shaving him all the time. I just kept watching how his barber did it and then I "experimented" on him.

I bought a regular plastic cape at a beauty supply store and a good pair of scissors; sat him down in front of the window to watch the birds and sang to him while I nervously cut his hair.

One positive here: you'll never be criticized for cutting his/her hair wrong. Your guy/gal will always be content with whatever you do. After a little practice I got pretty good; even if I do say so myself.

I really don't like cutting toenails. I feel sorry for anyone who has to make their living doing this. But you have to do what you have to do. Frank's toenails began getting thicker and thicker. This seems to be the norm for the elderly too. I ended up taking him occasionally to a podiatrist who sanded his thickened nails. This made it much easier for me to keep his toenails shortened.

Frank's doctor cautioned me to be sure to keep his fingernails short and blunt. (Patients with sensitive skin can scratch themselves and become infected.) Now I am very vigilante about keeping his nails clean and short. Filing used to drive him crazy before he became sick; but now I can file his nails after cutting them (making them smooth also helps with scratches.)

Concerning his teeth; Frank was always conscientious about brushing his teeth and regular cleaning appointments. After a few years, at a regular cleaning appointment the dentist told us he had two cavities! He never had cavities! The dentist suggested I take over his brushings. I discovered that he was running the electric toothbrush but not covering any of his teeth! He had forgotten how to brush! In his dentist's opinion- Frank's longer life was due to my consistent brushing of his teeth. Regular dental cleaning for him has made his breath smell sweeter and he's less prone to infections in other parts of his body. Score one for me!

I know, you'll be thinking: "This is just too much work." Just remember that nursing homes will not take the time to do as good a job on these things as you will. After all; you're doing this out of love; but for others it's just to make a living. Remember too, the more you do the care giving, the easier and less time consuming it will become. You'll develop your own unique skills and the satisfaction of a job well done.

Now go forth and "experiment"!

Frank's Clothes

Since you and your guy/gal is just now dealing with this disease, you may not even have to use this chapter. Remember I said the Doctors are very close to an early detection and treatment for most Dementia patients? Please read more about this in "The Last Chapter".

At first all his clothes were fine. After a while, especially after incontinence reared its ugly head; I looked for easier ways to change his clothes.

When I first began to dress Frank myself, I found it easier to buy elastic wasted pants and shorts. I also purchased some oversized polo shirts. (It is much easier on and off when the shirts are not form fitting.) Language is also important when dressing him/her. I ask him to lift his "arms to the ceiling when putting his shirts on or off. I also make a game of peek-a-boo when changing his shirts.

I kept one or two pairs of "good" pants and shirts for special occasions. I sewed huge heavy duty snaps instead of buttons at the top of the zippers. (Easier for me than buttons or grommets.)

As for shoes: I began to find that his loafers were easier than tied shoes or tennis shoes to put on him. I even found sandals that had Velcro straps in the backs. I cut the back out of one pair of shoes that became a "slip on pair".

Socks. Remember I said how sensitive their skin becomes? Well I found out the hard way when I discovered large red pressure patches on his shins. (This, after a few days of wearing his regular dress socks.) I realized it was the socks making his shins red. I bought diabetic socks for him and the red patches went away. I also bought one size larger socks and they worked fine too.

Even though Frank's skin is overly sensitive; he doesn't register pain the same way he used to.

One day (when he was still able to be trusted to ride his bike around the block AND come back, he was bitten by a pit bull!) He came home, showered and ate dinner. Later that evening he lifted his sweat pant leg saying: "I think this might need a band aide." I was shocked. Six inches of his right shin bone was showing through! I took him to the ER and they told me it was so serious that he might need a skin graph! Luckily for us his leg healed without the skin graph.

In my "wordy way" I just want you to be especially vigilant about any skin breaks or bruising. You just can't rely on your guy/gal to complain about pain.

I know, it's just one more thing to worry about! You CAN handle this.

"To Drive or Not To Drive"

Finding the right moment to start hiding the keys - literally- is going to be tough. Lucky for me in our state they have a law that requires doctors to report any diagnosis of Dementia or related brain diseases to the DMV.

A few months after our visits to San Francisco, a letter came from the DMV. It asked that Frank come in and be retested in order to drive a vehicle. We live 14 miles from the nearest town so it seemed unfair to "clip his wings" so soon.

After much studying and worrying; he passed his test. The next year he passed, just barely. He and I agreed that he wasn't to drive to town anymore; just to visit his sister and uncle a few miles away. This he did for a while. I did try to get him to ride his bike around our small ranch, just so he could feel freer. And I made time to drive him here and there for visits farther away.

On our ranch we have several ranch pickups, tractors, and such. All had keys, but I wasn't too worried. (I should have been.)

One day (before I had installed the child locks on all the outside doors) He drove away in one of the pickups. I was so scared! I called all of the relatives and friends I could think of. No one had seen him or his little blue pickup. After what seemed like hours he drove slowly back up the driveway. He said: "I just felt like having a mocha at Starbucks." (The nearest Starbucks is 35 miles away!) I was surprised he even found his way home!

After that the childproofing and hiding of ALL keys began!

Whenever he would ask why he wasn't driving, I told him that the DMV had pulled his license. (The following year we never even applied for a license for him.)

He still wants to drive. And once in a while he'll beat me into the driver's seat. I just very calmly urge him out, saying: "I can't let you drive. You don't have your license anymore."

This is a very hard thing for you to do. But for your safety and his/hers you must be firm. Some relatives even came up to me in later years telling me of near misses they had observed while he was driving alone! (I could have used that information when it was occurring!) So I guess you could say I dodged the bullet on that one. Be vigilante and strong for the both of you.

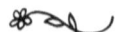

The First and Last Chapter

Can I tell you just a little of our beginning?

Frank and I met while we were both sophomores in different high schools. There was a college in our town. So when I was introduced to him I thought he was a "college man"! He was so grown up and serious and shy.

It was love at first sight for both of us. We dated until our graduations. That summer he gave me an engagement ring. We were engaged while I went to college and he worked with his father in rice farming. We married in 1961. He has always been the love of my life. We both felt lucky to have found our soul mates. It was a happy life. Of course there were tough times. Bumpy roads go with the wedded journey. But I wouldn't trade living in a small town and raising my children in a rural setting for any other life.

After 44 years of marriage to a healthy strong, never smoked, never drank, never overweight, workaholic farmer; I watched as he became more and more tired- "Walking in mud" was his description. Tests upon tests revealed a healthy heart and body. Finally a neurologist declared his brain was atrophying! His brain x-rays showed the brain of an 80 year old when he was only 61!

I was stunned. After several "second opinions" and much research on my part, I was lucky to have a friend in San Francisco who "walked" his medical history to the neurology department at UCSF. We had visited UC San Diego, for a second opinion and they told us that UCSF was doing the best research in this area. The doctors at UCSF invited Frank to become a research subject. And so it began 10 years ago.

We have gone back to UCSF each year for a hospital stay. The doctors and researchers examine him, test him, take blood samples (his DNA is in a "safe place") and will outlive all of us. They have even taken skin tissue from his thigh and turned it into stem cells and are successfully growing his brain cells in their labs! The doctors will have his brain to study after his death.

All this, in the feverish effort to find a treatment and any early detection test.

Most of the doctors agree that Dementia begins much earlier than current tests reveal. Frank has done many tests for early detection and various experimental drugs, to slow the Dementia. None have worked so far.

But there is hope. Maybe not for Frank and me, but in the next few years I believe they will find a "cure" and or treatment.

Do not despair, the doctors are so dedicated and work such long hours with limited funds and in such small compact spaces- they are really determined to help us.

Frank is still here at home. I know there will come a time when I will no longer have the strength to care for him by myself. But I am determined to keep him with me for as long as I possibly can.

Please do not blame yourself when the time comes that you need to have others care for him/her in a nursing home. I know this will be a guilt filled, heart wrenching decision. Just remember to love, love for as long, long, long as you can. Do not let anyone make you feel guilty. No one can know the pull of such decisions unless they have had to do this themselves. Be strong.

Meanwhile use your brain and the individual skills only you have, to "stay on the path God has chosen for you." (After all we <u>both</u> know WE wouldn't chose this journey for ourselves!)

Questions and Answers

1. <u>How do I remember all the "stuff" in this book?</u>
    A. One day at a time. When I started care giving in earnest 6 years ago, I knew nothing. Frank's decline has been slow motion and I learned little by little. My only goal then and now, is to keep him healthy, clean and safe for as long as I possibly can. Just take it "one day at a time".

2. <u>How can I cope with all these feelings I have- guilt, grief, fear, anger, etc.?</u>
    A. It helps to have a strong faith. Just knowing this is a journey you wouldn't in a million years want for yourself- and having faith that God is keeping track- will get you stronger and farther on your journey. If you have lost touch with your faith, now is the time to talk to someone of the clergy. He can help you "get your head on straight"! Uh-oh-preaching, sorry!

3. <u>I feel like I want to end it all right now! How do I cope?</u>

A. That's understandable. You'll have these thoughts from time to time. More at first, less as time passes. Just know that within you is a strong person fighting to come out. Time will make you stronger. I also tell myself, after a day of this negative stuff has come and gone: "I was really in a funk, missed too much sleep, not eating right, need to get over myself and get on with my reason for being here: Frank!"

4. <u>I am so jealous and sad when I see other couples together laughing and happy and healthy. What can I do?</u>

A. I have been there too. After a while, I learned to just look at them and be happy for them. I don't let my envy pull me down. I have learned that for me- grief, envy, fear, are just too taxing for me to keep in my head! Those strong feelings just drain me emotionally and physically. I have learned to nip them before they stay in my head. (Just in one ear and out the other.)

5. <u>What do Dementia and Alzheimer's patients die from?</u>

A. I have asked myself this many times. Even the doctors are vague about this. Keeping your loved one healthy is part of a long life for anyone.

Flu, pneumonia, car accidents we all die from something. I think the doctors just don't know and maybe that's just as well for us. I just count myself lucky for each day with Frank and am continually surprised at the end of each one. You will have more questions. I can't think of any now. But you will. That's why I recommend that you find an Alzheimer's group as soon as you can. They will have answers for you. Don't let shyness or any another excuse keep you from doing this. And don't wait too long. (I Did.)

After His Fall

Do not, I repeat do not read this chapter until you are SURE that your loved one has reached the very last stages of this sad disease! You should not see, in this chapter, your future. It may not be this way for you.

Your experience will be different than mine. It should be: your history and strengths will be different also. My guy was nine years into his FTD. He had not spoken or uttered a word for more than a year. He was losing weight. (No matter that he ate everything I put before him; in between meal snacks, yogurt, ice cream, anything fattening, I could think of.)

And still, he was skin with bones underneath, just wasting away.

He could still take simple directions like closing a drawer or holding an object. And he could still give me a kiss when I asked! He was still strong enough to do his daily "walk abouts", around the kitchen table.

From my earlier chapters, I told you we had a three level house on a ranch 30 miles from any doctors, drugstores, ETC. I always knew I would sell the ranch and move to a one story house. But I figured it would be after Frank died. Little did I know God had a different plan for me.

One day an old high school pal of Frank's came to my door. He had become a real-estate agent and he had an offer for me. I heard him out, telling him I had been advised to never sell my land. But, his visit had me thinking: Why would I want to be the third widow on my country road? (Women in my area tend to stay years and years after their husbands are gone.) Why shouldn't I want to sell my house and move to a town nearer Frank's doctors, skilled nurses, a house with one story, where Frank would be safer?

God must have been planning this all along! Because within two months, I had sold my ranch house, found a cute smaller house in the town I grew up in, moved (more about this later) and I was back to my caregiving routine: with Frank doing his "walk abouts" around the same dining room table! He had adjusted beautifully to his new surroundings!

Bless his heart, he waited until we were settled (boxes put away) to walk, walk, walk, then shuffle, shuffle, shuffle; slowly slumping against the dining room wall. (He had become unable to stand or use his arms to eat). Friends thought he had had a stroke. Frank's doctors said this sometimes happens when the brain is not telling the muscles what to do. Then I remembered: two years before, the research doctors at UCSF had remarked how well he was walking. (They'd expected his abilities in this area to be markedly diminished even at that time.)

★★★★★★★★★★★

And so...... my new challenges to Frank's caregiving began. It was laughter and tears on my part; big widened eyes when I messed up on his part. My comments to him were things like: "it's OK, Frank- try not to be scared- but I'd be scared if someone like me was just learning how to move you from the hospital bed to your wheel chair in this thing!"

Because Frank could no longer help me, I had to have a "Hoyer lift" delivered along with a hospital bed (Make sure the bed has a motorized head and legs – extra money-but more than worth it!)

About the Hoyer Lift: It's a chrome triangular device with a hydraulic hand pump that enables the caregiver to (with a properly placed sling under the patient) lift him out of bed and into a wheel chair or recliner. A great invention; but one I looked upon as a "torture device"! Make sure when the rental deliveryman comes, that he actually puts your loved one in the sling and lifts and places him in a bed, chair, ECT. I mistakenly thought I could do this using the instruction book that came with it. Mistake! It is dangerous for you, the caregiver, and for the patient, to use this lift without the proper training. Don't depend on any CNA to know! The, best, safest method, is to have it demonstrated TO you. Frank and I were lucky. I didn't drop him! (We had some interesting adventures-one where I had him upside down!) He soon trusted me enough that he would fall asleep while I transported him down the hall!

A great friend (recently widowed) lent me her husband's fancy wheel chair. I became knowledgeable about calling the local medical transport company to help transport him, in his wheel chair, to his important doctor and dental appointments.

I was exhausted. But I knew, from my past, that once I had learned all these new challenging skills, I would get into my "time and effort mode" and things would get easier. And they did!

I was able to have people come for a few hours, three times a week. The local Home Health CNAs gave him better bed baths than I could. I also bought a ringed "shampoo kit" that allowed me to wash his hair while he was in the hospital bed. I learned valuable tips from each of the different CNAs. They had little shortcuts to his care. Each one had a different approach, and method. I used their ideas to create my own personalized care for Frank.

When I bought this little house I had had in mind giving Frank a shower in the huge walk in shower. But the wheeled shower chair could not safely wheel him over its two inch threshold. My handy man made a hinged wooden ramp to fit over the threshold. I could then (with help from a CNA) wheel Frank into the shower and give him a thorough bath once a week.

I bought a large plastic apron from a beauty supply store and pinned it in back to protect my clothes while I gave him his shower with a handheld shower wand. I tried to get the bathroom as warm as I could and used three big bath towels to dry him. I had the CNA standby to help me get him out once he was dry. I also kept two or three plastic bags in the shower for "little accidents" during his showers. You'll get the hang of it after a few tries.

It's amazing to me how easily we can all adapt given time; to the changing circumstances of our lives. My belief in God and His Son Jesus has helped me through this scary time. OK, enough preaching, already!

Frank's last "walk about" happened in the Fall of the year- a mere ten days after I brought him home to the new little house. (I had decided that he would be safer and less scared if he wasn't around when the movers came to pack up the house we had lived in for 38 years.) I found a facility whose staff knew him. I arranged for him to stay for ten days while I moved and unpacked and tried to have all his familiar surroundings the same as they were in the old house.

Don't be afraid to move if you need to: downsizing was hard but doable and really did me a world of good. The things you find that are dear to you are not so dear to your family. Just asking and letting them know you are making these choices allows your family to be open about the things they would like. It's surprisingly helpful for the future and you won't have to save all this "stuff" no one wants!

For instance my mother's piano: (so beloved and played by her) was to go to her only granddaughter, who never learned to play. After discussing it, she was OK with my giving it to a family friend who had been a catechism student years ago and who played beautifully. It was a win-win since I couldn't take it with me to the smaller house.

I found things I had forgotten I had. It felt strange to leave the past behind, but as I gave away Frank's and my things from the past it felt right. I made a point of giving things to people I knew would want them and use them. I was careful to feel out the recipients so they wouldn't feel pressured into taking something they didn't really want. And, added bonus, Frank adjusted wonderfully; as though he had always lived in this little house!

★★★★★★★★

Should I tell you about the day he died? I don't want you to be sad. It's was so how I wanted his life to end: loved, and with me holding him.

He developed a high fever (103 degrees) in just a few minutes. One moment I was washing his face to begin our day. I left his hospital bed to prepare his breakfast, came back; he was flushed, perspiring, with that high fever. I made him as comfortable as possible, with alcohol rubs, crushed Tylenol and ice chips. He seemed to rally on the next day. A nurse who examined him said: "He had diminished lung sounds." She said his body was doing what it should do to fight this off. I concentrated on keeping him comfortable. Although somewhere in the back of my mind; I realized this might only be the first in a series of illnesses. I didn't want to think about that. I just wanted to comfort him and tell him I loved him and not to be afraid.

After rallying in the morning of the second day; he took a turn for the worse that night. He was having a very hard time taking each breath. I kept him hydrated by giving him ice chips and letting them melt in his mouth. (At this point he was too weak to use a straw or swallow from a cup.) I should note, I was in contact with his local doctor all during this time.

When something hits me (memories I guess) my stomach knots and I feel the loss of Frank. But I know that I can choose to remember the sadness or let it go. I just don't dwell on these feelings. I refuse to let painful, guilty feelings turn me into the weak crying person I used to be.

Frank always had a great sense of timing. He was always on time even early, for appointments.

Over the years he influenced me to make this a priority; sometimes by example other times by chastising me. He continued this "timing" even to his last day:

Scheduling for CNAs was done a week in advance. His fever had developed over the weekend. So that morning when the CNA showed up, I went out to the bank and market. When I came back, I sent her home and I sat by his bed, giving him ice chips and alcohol rubs. He could have died any time while I was out; but he waited; waited until I returned.

He was so weak and dripping perspiration. I was changing the wet absorbent pad under his shoulders, he was so limp. I put my arms around him and I asked him for a kiss. He gave me a kiss! Thinking back now I am convinced he knew me. (He didn't kiss anybody but me.)

I whispered in his ear "it's OK to go. Don't be afraid. Look for your mom and dad and our little grandson Grant." At that point he stopped making those loud sounds when he breathed. It was quiet in the room. I closed his eyes. He was with Jesus. I knew I had done my best; but now had to continue with the plans for his transport to the funeral home, arrange for the autopsy team to come from San Francisco to harvest his brain for their studies. All the calls were right there on my list and I focused on those tasks at hand. That list was my salvation during those next few minutes!

A few weeks before, my dear friend (who visited me regularly and sometimes watched Frank while I went to the market) asked me to write down the phone calls she would have to make if Frank died suddenly while I was away. This was the best suggestion! That list was a blessing!

I had to inquire from his doctor the best steps and numbers to call. I even wrote down the words to say upon calling those numbers. I posted them by the phone and made a copy for my desk. I attached the list next to the names of people and numbers I had compiled months ago for relatives and friends to call when Frank died.

That little list helped me get through those first few hours, as I called. That list kept me calm and focused. Make a list.

★★★★★★★★★★★★

I know others have loved as much as I. Others have struggled more. Others have expressed their journeys more beautifully.

I only know that Frank is with me always, in all I do. I know I did my best and will not allow regrets to shadow my memories of the joy we shared for 53 years. I would not change any of the days God laid out for Frank and me.

Something I have only recently learned: You will never truly know when you have followed God's path for you until you can look back at the choices you have made and see the pattern of His guidance. When you can do that, then you will know.